KICK NICOTINE

Vaping, Smoking, Chewing

Fast and Free and Lose Weight Doing It

Immediate Results

DOUG EWALD

PAGE PUBLISHING, INC.
New York, NY

First originally published by Page Publishing, Inc. 2019

ISBN 978-1-64544-126-7 (Paperback)
ISBN 978-1-64544-127-4 (Digital)

Printed in the United States of America

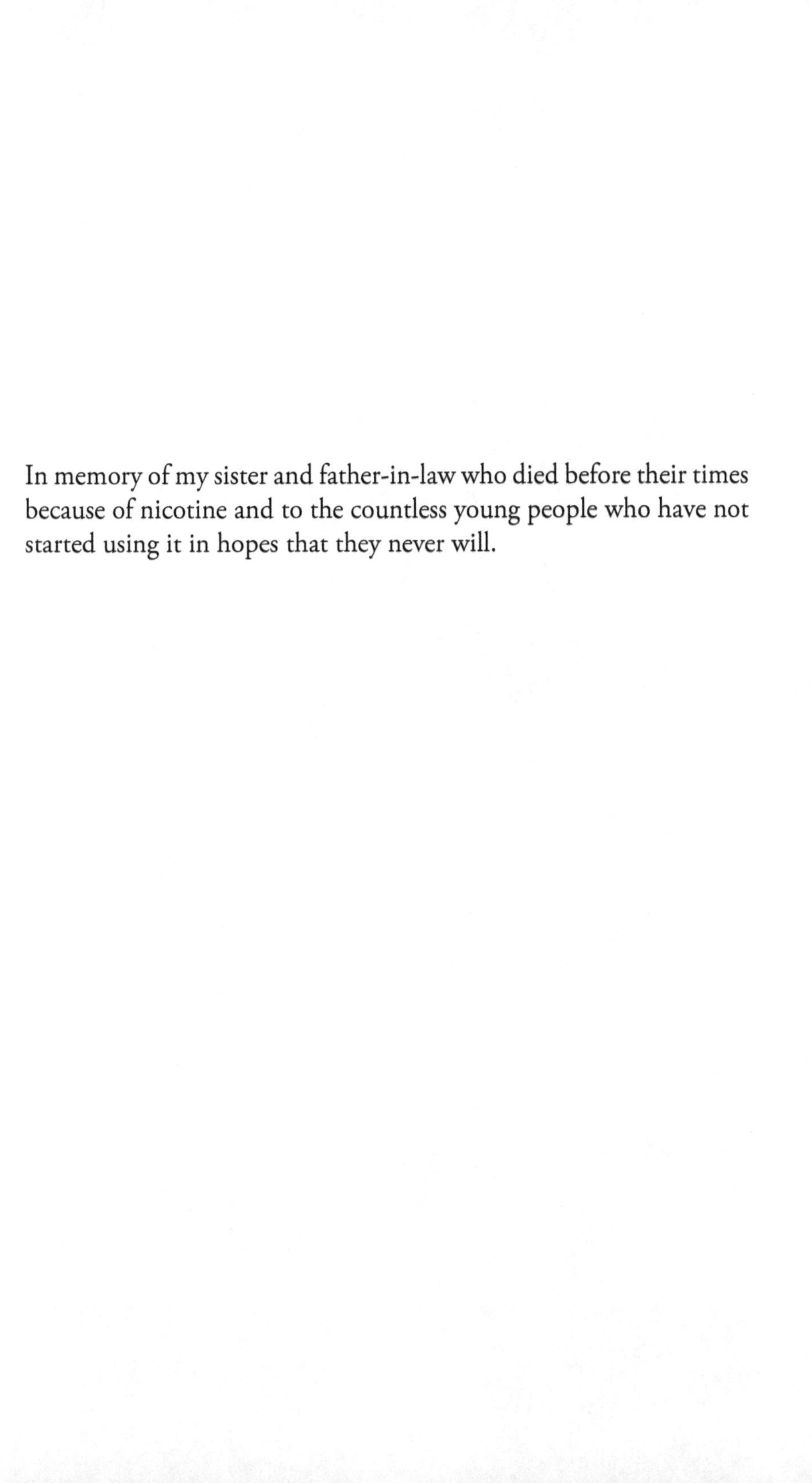
In memory of my sister and father-in-law who died before their times because of nicotine and to the countless young people who have not started using it in hopes that they never will.

Age forty-two, sixty pounds overweight, continuously coughing and sick. Tried quitting many times unsuccessfully, each time followed by weight gain. Goal: one final attempt at quitting must be successful; failure, not an option. An immediate miracle was needed before a health catastrophe.

Here are the simple steps that succeeded.

Preface

This booklet was originally written and published to help smokers quit smoking. The ensuing years have shown, however, that addressing smoking only was missing a sizeable part of the target when the real enemy should have been identified as nicotine abuse in any of its many forms.

Nicotine is a vicious, dangerous drug thought by many experts to be as addictive and habit forming as heroin. While public awareness of the dangers of nicotine has increased, its usage is increasing, particularly among younger people.

The industries that grow, process, and sell tobacco, and thus nicotine, spend countless millions to discover new markets and methods of selling their product. Again, younger people are singled out as more impressionable and likely to jump aboard the nicotine train because "everyone is doing it," and they have a lot of time ahead of them to quit.

Unfortunately, the human brain is not totally developed until the mid-twenties and much irreversible damage can be done by nicotine use prior to that age.

You can spend a lot of money to kick an addiction to nicotine, and it's easy to say that it's worth any expense to do so. Of course, health is the overall most important reason to quit, but the expenses involved in the addiction must be considered as well. You will find no end to the professional services, products, and procedures available to help nicotine users kick their habit from very inexpensive to the unbelievably expensive. Some are successful; others aren't. Some of the products developed to assist users in quitting even contain nicotine itself! Some services will walk with you for the rest of your life to help you stay away from nicotine.

You needn't spend much money at all to quit nicotine use. You are the only person who can decide which route to take, and the decision boils down to the very simple question: Can you control your own mind?

Can you control your own mind? As simple as it sounds, the answer to this question determines how you should go about defeating the enemy—nicotine addiction. It's not an easy question to answer, and there is no right or wrong response; the important thing is to get on with whatever you decide to do.

Your own mind can be your best friend or worst enemy at times, as you've probably found out in your life already. Please don't hesitate to admit that you would rather not put your mind to the test and seek whatever assistance you might need in getting nicotine out of your life.

Giving up nicotine is neither easy nor difficult, depending on how you look at it. In my case, there was no pain, but there was a lot of self-doubt and anguish—for a short time. The most surprising memory I have is how little time it really took: at the end of the first day, there was the pride of arriving at that point. Three days into the "quit" was the awareness of how much easier it came for me to breathe, and my sense of smell and taste improved.

This very short book will not remove nicotine from your life. Hopefully, it will give you some moral support, encouragement, and ideas that will speed you along your way to a new life free of nicotine and the countless problems that come along with it. This is one of the more efficient methods of nicotine cessation: you decide to do it, you do it, and you're done—no meetings, no medications, no fees. Just get it done!

My Story

My nicotine abuse started so simply: a fishing trip to northern Minnesota with my best buddy to celebrate the end of our freshman year in college. While stopping to gas up on the way home, the sight of some cigarettes by the cashier prompted a spontaneous question: "Hey, Jon, why don't we start smoking?" Jon's agreement started a nicotine-related dependence of twenty-three years.

Although the initial nicotine "carrier" was a cigarette, pipes, and cigars soon followed, and even a brief "chaw" of snuff. Had the nicotine industry thought of vaping at the time, it would have been part of the menu as well.

During the three-hour drive home, the habit became an essential part of my life although cough inducing, foul smelling, and bad tasting, as well as expensive. Well, over $200,000 in today's prices was spent "enjoying" the addiction that resulted in innumerable headaches, dozens of severe bouts with bronchitis, chest colds, and one hospitalization.

Friends and relatives continually informed me that quitting nicotine use leads to weight gain so, of course, I believed them. Even though I made many attempts to quit "using" nicotine, not only were none successful but also each effort resulted in sizeable weight gains. My normal weight increased by sixty pounds because of the fear that giving up nicotine would lead to weight gain.

It wasn't just my body that paid the price. Over the years, my wife and children were continually bathed in a toxic atmosphere, and our home reeked of tobacco. Suits, shirts, ties, jackets, slacks, and one whole car seat succumbed. Add to the list a few table cloths and carpet burns as well.

There was not one good, positive thing that could be said about the drug that held me so close except, perhaps, that it felt so wonderful when giving into the urge to use after another failed attempt to quit.

My sister died of lung cancer in her sixties from smoking. My father-in-law passed away at age seventy from emphysema, now grouped with other similar afflictions under the umbrella of COPD. In the closing moments of his life, the hospital nurse in attendance looked at his family as we stood around his bed and said, "After seeing this, please don't ever start smoking."

After twenty-three years of nicotine use, it would not have been wrong to refer to me as a "health time bomb."

Grossly overweight at 232 pounds, smoking sixty cigarettes per day and afraid to quit for fear of gaining even more weight, my life was in need of a miracle.

Essentially I had a permanent "cold" that consisted of continual coughing and recurrent spells of severe chest pain when coughing. The pain was so great one night; upon visiting a hospital emergency room, I was immediately hospitalized and was relieved to find out the next morning that it was "only" severe bronchitis.

At this point, having tried unsuccessfully to quit my addiction to nicotine countless times it occurred to me that perhaps I could find a new, healthier addiction that could help me replace nicotine. A miracle was needed, and it was needed soon: not only did nicotine need to leave my life but fifty plus pounds needed to go with it.

No one could have ever referred to me as an athlete, and aerobic activities were so painful over the years that once tried, they were soon quit. But the distance running craze was in its early phases, and eventually, the idea of becoming a runner entered my mind. My reasoning was that if the horrid idea of running could be overcome, and if it could ever become enjoyable, it just could become the healthy replacement for nicotine. It might even help make nicotine use less enjoyable. And it just might result in weight loss too.

Addicted to LSD

My apologies to Timothy Leary, but one of the buzz phrases that accompanied the early running craze particularly appealed to me because the benefits of this sport were thought to best be realized through Long Slow Distances and lots of it.

My goal was to become a LSD runner, and all that was needed was a plan.

Let me briefly explain the concept of winter in Minnesota: the days in the R months are cold here, and the nights are even colder. My plan was to drop nicotine on New Year's Eve and to start my running career on November 1—sixty-one days earlier. My running would be done secretively under the cover of night—outside. No one, not even my wife or children would be aware of what was going on; "out for a walk" was the adequate explanation for my absence.

After dinner on the night of November 1 when all family members were otherwise involved, my running career began. My first running goal was to make it between two consecutive telephone poles by a flat street in our neighborhood. No street lights. And no smoking while running. Or what I called running.

My lungs were so congested that the halfway mark between those two telephone poles instantly became a mid-November goal. And that first drag on my post run cigarettes in the blackness of a Minnesota November night was instant pain. It took real determination to enjoy that sensation.

What a pathetic sight there must have been on that street that night! A hulk of a man hiding from the world while attempting to look and act like a runner. But falling asleep was enhanced by a new sensation: it had to be pride because the first step toward my goal had been taken. Eventually, the world would have a new runner and ex-nicotine user.

Around the first of December, the news was broken to my wife and our children: January 1 was to be the first day of the rest of my life as a non-nicotine user. It was kind of a pledge made to those who meant the most to me and also a solicitation of their patience and understanding during what was expected to be a trying time. But there had been trying times before, and they had all ended after days of pain and suffering by giving in to demon nicotine and the nervous weight gain that followed.

On December 15, I dropped my longtime favorite brand of smokes and started using another far less favorite. But the new ones "delivered the goods" even if they didn't taste as good as the old "cancer sticks." As many of the world's great accomplishments have been made because of small details, it seemed that my major goal would also rest on smaller precedent details and perhaps changing from a favorite brand to a less favorite one just before quitting might just help.

That very day, as if by Divine Guidance, the memory of a smoking experiment carried out thirteen years earlier came to mind. It is detailed here because this experiment became the backbone of my final successful attempt to kick nicotine.

The Experiment

Seven years into my nicotine nightmare, a miracle occurred, but it took sixteen more years before it was realized. Here's what happened.

My older brother shared an office with me in our family business. We were both smokers who worked with a large number of others, many of whom shared our addiction. One day, a salesman challenged me to bet a dollar on a simple experiment. The challenge was that it was impossible to tell whether or not a cigarette was lighted if you couldn't see it or smell it or feel it.

They placed me in front of, but facing away from, a large floor fan, which was turned on so that smoke from lighted cigarettes could not reach my nose.

Then my brother put a hefty blindfold over my eyes so that there was no chance of me seeing. And ten of my brand of cigarettes were placed between my lips one at a time for inhaling—some lighted and some not.

My thumbs up signaled that I thought the current cigarette was lighted, and thumbs down that it wasn't.

The experiment ended and proved my ability to discern whether or not a cigarette was lighted: my judgment was right six out of ten times! Smugly, I pocketed the two dollars and onlookers agreed with my smoke detecting acumen.

What was significant but not realized until sixteen years later upon my making the decision to give up nicotine once and for all was that I could not tell by inhaling and holding a puff whether or not a cigarette was lighted 40 percent of the time!

This minor detail remembered by accident just two weeks before my "final assault" made my most difficult early quitting days much easier.

The detail, simply stated is: if I could only guess correctly 60 percent of the time whether or not a cigarette was lighted or not, then nearly half the time, there must be a similar effect from just taking a good deep breath of pure, fresh nicotine-free air and holding it as long as possible.

The final two weeks of my nicotine-polluted life were spent in planning the three weeks that would follow them and repeated long-held deep breaths.

Starting the New Year as a non-nicotine user made sense because it was the busiest time of my life. I had three concurrent jobs at the time, and add to that, the time that needed to be spent with my wife and six children, and there wasn't a lot of time to be spent on a bad habit.

It occurred to me that a slogan might be helpful—something that could be repeated over and over again in self—talk to speed me along the way. And so the slogan or mantra that became my battle cry was:

> "I don't want it, I don't need it, and I'm not going
> to do it!" With that and a couple of deep breaths,
> a guy could almost conquer a kingdom…

> Cigarettes is a curse on the whole human race; a
> man is a monkey with one in his face. Here is my
> definition believe me dear brother: a fire on one
> end and a fool on the other!

These words to a song written by Nashville songwriter Tim Spencer in 1947 captivated me because of my long-held opinion of how dumb my reflection in store windows looked with a cigarette sticking out of my face. So I began paying close attention to smokers and their actions: people paying after-tax money to make themselves sick and look stupid—including me. Would I hire that person in the reflection or want to see one of our kids dating him or her?

My mind was totally aware of how difficult it would be to once-and-for-all quit, but it also remembered that the truly tough times, the first three days, had been surpassed many times.

Another mantra: Quit once for good, and the tough times are done forever.

Who was in charge of *my* life—tobacco company executives who probably wouldn't hire heavy smokers because of their illness and/or absentee rates or *me*? If I am in charge, then I'd better get going.

One thing to do for certain is to take the actual amount of cash that would go into nicotine usage each day and stash it away. The first purchase when there was enough cash in the sock was a brand-new pair of Nike Daybreak running shoes, size 12.

My last two weeks were dedicated to finding all nicotine-related products and gear and putting everything in one box. Lighters, matches, breath mints (the only people they fooled were the smokers anyway), lighter flints and fluid, pipe tobacco pouches, pipe cleaners and tools, and more. All would be disposed of on D-Day minus one by placing all materials in a waterproof garbage bag, covering the whole collection with pancake syrup to eliminate the temptation to revisit it, and trashing the whole mess.

I started to compile a list of all former nicotine users whom I knew and respected. This was a real help because not only were these people I respected, but the longer the list got, the more I realized that there are an awful lot of former smokers who have successfully walked the trail that would soon be in front of me. And if that many people have already quit, could it be that it's really that tough to do once you make your mind up to it?

My mind could, at times, be my worst enemy, capable of saying things like: "Poor you, having to give up something you really love and want to do. And when you can quit whenever you want, it's too bad you have to give up one of your freedoms. And look at all those people who are smoking and having a good time." It became an interesting challenge to deal with those thoughts; I found that changing what I was doing was the best way to get them out of my mind.

I did some financial planning in those last two weeks. As a three-pack-a-day smoker, it was simple math to round off my annual purchases as one thousand packs of smokes. That started to run into money! Think of that in terms of today's prices.

And all of that money for what? No, it's not for nothing—that would be a far better outcome than what you really are getting for your money that, in reality, is nothing but negatives, some of which have you ending up dead. Really no-coming-back, no-second- chance *dead*.

Think of it. Gasping for breath, wheezing, unable to get around, coughing up blood *dead*. Think of people crying at funerals; children losing parents who could have prevented it all, it should be called suicide because when you use nicotine willfully, that's really what it is.

Vaping and Other Nicotine Delivery Systems

Vaping is the newest phenomenon in the nicotine delivery systems parade. Vaping utilizes a battery operated heating system by which nicotine dissolved in a usually attractively flavored liquid, is then vaporized, and the vapor inhaled by the user. A wide variety of such devices may be purchased (fifty dollars for a starter kit!) to send usually younger future users on their merry way to nicotine addiction. A recent full-page ad in the Minneapolis *Star Tribune* states that their cartridges contain "a salt based e-liquid to satisfy smokers when transitioning away from cigarettes."

The same ad includes the following statements:

> WARNING: This product contains nicotine. Nicotine is an addictive chemical.

And at the very bottom of the ad these words:

> IF YOU DON'T SMOKE OR VAPE, DON'T START.

The public menace is not smoking, chewing, or vaping; it is nicotine or any product that contains it.

In December 2016, the US Surgeon General issued a groundbreaking report "E-Cigarette Use Among Youth and Young Adults" that made a number of important conclusions and findings about the use of e-cigarettes among youth. These included that the flavors in e-cigarettes are one of the main reasons youth use them, e-cigarette aerosol is not safe and that e-cigarette use is strongly associated with the use of other tobacco products among youth and young adults.

Most importantly, the Surgeon General concluded that e-cigarette use among youth is now a significant public health concern and steps must be taken by parents, educators, and especially policymakers to discourage use of e-cigarettes.

A special warning to young people and their parents:

If you are under the age of twenty-five years, or if you are the parents, relatives, or friends of anyone in that age range, please do some research before using or allowing to use nicotine in any form. The scientific literature is exhaustive on the potential lifelong negative effects of nicotine use particularly in this age range.

It is common knowledge that some parents and children actually consider vaping as a miracle tool to prevent future tobacco use; such thinking is absolutely and totally wrong.

Any use of nicotine, certainly including vaping, will in a very short time lead to nicotine dependence, and in young people, this can have life-threatening implications far outweighing useless costs of the habit.

Finally, a subtle danger in vaping is that the attractiveness and taste of the flavorings used in the liquid makes it extremely dangerous, and easy, particularly in individuals under the age of twenty five years of age, to overdose on nicotine.

Further, the health and scientific communities are becoming increasingly concerned about the frequency of seizures among young 'vapers'. The potential implications here are serious enough that users and their families should consider discontinuing the practice.

Certainly the best way to avoid nicotine addiction is to never start its use.

Nicotine the Drug

Nicotine belongs to the stimulant family of drugs; it occurs naturally in a variety of plants, most notably in tobacco and is responsible for its addictive property. As a stimulant, it is known to speed bodily functions and cause users to experience temporary feelings of increased energy and vitality. Because it constricts blood vessels, it may cause insomnia causing users to feel more alert at first.

Although it is a highly addictive drug, it is still legal to purchase and use nicotine in the United States with certain age restrictions. An increasing number of states and municipalities are attempting to regulate its purchase and use by younger users—those most susceptible to its addictive properties.

Nicotine need not be smoked to be effective. It is extremely addictive whether smoked, chewed, or inhaled from an electronic device. It is frequently added to weight-loss remedies, energy-enhancing products, and even in some products advertised as aids in smoking cessation.

The use of nicotine leads to myriad health-related problems including, but not limited, to the following:

> Appearance changes: including wrinkles and sallow complexion
> Adolescent brain development implications
> Cancer in multiple sites
> Cataracts and macular degeneration
> Chronic bronchitis, other respiratory problems
> Diabetes

Emphysema
Gastric complications, ulcers, and indigestion
Heart disease, multiple types
Leukemia
Oral and dental diseases including cancer
Pregnancy complications
Sensory loss, particularly taste, smell stroke

Businesses selling nicotine are continually seeking new ways for individuals to buy and use it. Countless millions of dollars on research has allowed the nicotine industry to develop creative new opportunities for consumer nicotine addiction such as vaping and related methods of use known as ENDS or "electronic nicotine delivery systems."

There are other entities in our society that are highly dependent on the success of the nicotine selling industry, surprising though they may be.

Pharmaceutical companies realize incalculable income from the sale of products developed and sold to assist consumers in stopping the use of nicotine. Some of these products even contain the very drug they are designed to combat—nicotine!

It is not difficult to find commercial courses and classes targeting nicotine use cessation.

Although it is possible to find such opportunities offered by agencies at no, or little, cost to the consumer, quite the opposite is true also. Although it might be said that it is worth any price to quit successfully, as a potential buyer, it will be wise to be wary.

It is generally known that units of government (local, state, and federal) exact taxes on the purchase of nicotine containing products; the total take by all governments is overwhelming. Tobacco taxes, called by lawmakers "sin taxes," are relatively easy to add to or increase via legislation being considered for passage. And constituents who are ex- or non-nicotine users are far less likely to complain as such taxes go up.

The health risks associated with nicotine use are difficult to enumerate but easy to understand when one realizes that nicotine is an easily addictive poison in small doses.

No human health condition is enhanced by the use of nicotine, and no one is unaffected: human nicotine use in all its forms has a serious negative effect on healthy living. Think back to those first minutes, hours, and days of your own nicotine addiction to help realize how it has affected your life.

Nicotine use is thought to be as addictive as the use of heroin or cocaine and discontinuing its use as difficult.

So vaping and the e-cigarette have made nicotine use much safer, right? Let's make one thing perfectly and totally clear: it is not just the act of smoking that is extremely dangerous; it is nicotine use in any way or form that is.

Although the act of inhaling tobacco smoke into one's lungs brings in a host of chemicals (and therefore other concerns) in addition to nicotine, it is the use of the addictive drug nicotine that must end.

Your Story

William Ernest Henley wrote the famous words: "I am the master of my fate. I am the captain of my soul."

And there's a message there for you—the only person in the world who will write your story, and like it or not, each day is being entered, permanently and unchangeably in that history. Who's in charge of your mind, your fate, your soul? Kicking nicotine is one of the rare situations where quitters always win.

My goal is to help you live your remaining days as a person who has dealt with and overcome the challenge of nicotine abuse; the use of any amount of nicotine in any form and at any time constitutes "abuse." It may or may not help you to know this, but countless millions of your fellow people have done it and are doing just fine, thank you. Breaking news: you can too.

Before we go any further, please do us both a favor and give some serious thought to answering the following questions:

1. What has been your life's greatest, most significant accomplishment to date? Think of your school days, athletic endeavors, family- and work-related events: What is it that took your best work, concentration, and determination in order to succeed? The energy involved in nicotine cessation can't compare with any of these, or the length of time involved.

2. What has been the most difficult feat you have accomplished in your life so far—finishing school, building a garage, overcoming illness, military service? Only you can

identify what it was that took your most diligent effort to complete. Again, while you, as I did, may someday be able to say that kicking nicotine was the toughest thing you've ever done, you'll be surprised to find out how short lived it really was.

3. What was your most memorable trip that you'll never forget? Your honeymoon, summiting Wyoming's Cloud Peak, band, choir or team trips anywhere could qualify. How you planned so carefully and looked forward to these days. Now think back: How quickly has the time gone by since your trip ended? How quickly did the trip itself seem to fly by? That's exactly how quickly the time will pass in your early days of kicking the habit! It is difficult for me to believe that I quit nearly forty years ago, and I've never looked back.

4. Who is or are the most important person or people in your life? Spouse, children, parents, family, friends—more than one of these? They are the ones who count the most—who are closest to you. And I'm betting that when you tell them what you're about to, you'll get their wholehearted support and encouragement.

5. Where does alcohol use fit into your daily life? Some people can take it or leave it and others can't. In many cases a drink or two helps to remove inhibitions and if this is your situation it would be very wise to set the use of alcohol aside in the early days of your nicotine cessation.

That's it. Take all the time you need to address each of the above and write them down if you'd like. The fun thing is that no one needs to know any of your answers, but they will become extremely important to you throughout the rest of your life.

Understand Your Problem

You voluntarily became addicted to the abuse of a dangerous drug, nicotine, that is threatening your life, sucking up your financial resources (all after taxes have been paid, by the way), and is obnoxious to everyone around you except other addicts and those selling you your drug.

Determine that you're going to quit.

You don't have to do this, you know—it's voluntary. But so was the decision to start using nicotine in the first place. Sure, that vaping starter kit only cost you fifty dollars or that first pack of cigarettes only ten dollars, but who was to think that those expenses were not only ongoing but going higher each day or month or year?

Why is it that you want to quit? Here are some of the best reasons:

Just for the health of it. You have a monster by the tail, and it will get the best of you, sooner or later. It's really ugly to watch someone literally cough themselves to death with lung cancer or emphysema. I saw it happen to my sister and father-in-law. Is there some rational reason why you think you may be immune from the effects of nicotine?

The cost of it. That fifty dollar starter kit seemed to evaporate, and you have to keep on buying the stuff. Fifty cents for a cigarette? Are you kidding me or not—and you have to keep buying them. Pardon me, but that runs into money that you might be able to use for something better.

The "obnoxiousness" of it. Take some time and watch people who are smoking, chewing, or vaping. Seriously, have you ever seen anything that looks (and is) so stupid? That you pay for?

There are so many reasons you should quit, and you know 'em all. While you're at it, think of all the reasons why you should keep using: that won't take much space.

Pick a Date to Quit.

Give yourself some time here, but not a lot. How about the first of the next month. Or the first of the year (if it's December). In short, why not get on with it—your habit's getting more ingrained, you're spending horrible amounts of money, and you're not improving your health, so just plainly *do it*! Do you have days coming when you wouldn't be able to use nicotine? Use them to your advantage and plan your start date just ahead of them.

Tell Your VIPs.

Tell those important people you identified in the fourth question as being most important. Don't be afraid to ask for their help, patience, and understanding. If they are non- or ex-nicotine users, and they are so important to you, your efforts will be met with joy and support. If they are currently "using," don't bother to tell them. Really, if we're both hooked on something terrible, why would I want you to quit and leave me hanging out there alone?

See Your Doctor.

Never a bad idea. You're going to make an abrupt change in the way you treat your heart, lungs, and countless other body parts, and it's always a good idea to let your doctor in on your plans. Ask if she or he approves of your quitting—let me know if they don't. While you're at it, ask if it would be smart for you to substitute a daily walk or run for your nicotine addiction. Or some other form of aerobic activity.

Remember this: the only people who gain weight when they quit using caffeine are those who tell themselves they will.

Avoid Users.

As mentioned above, particularly in the early days and weeks of your "quitting," the less time you spend with users, the better. Don't seek opportunities to be with users and avoid them when possible. It just might be that greatest thing you have in common with some of your friends is that you are all users. Stop and think: Is a friendship based on the fact that you both share the same drug addiction something to base a long-term friendship on? You just may be better off without those friends.

Embrace Quitters.

Having given up nicotine will open up a whole new arena full of friends: those who have gone before you. Don't be afraid to ask them how they did it. This kind of quitter is always happy to share their secrets with you.

Prepare Your Own Mind.

Your best friend or your worst, dealing with your own mind can make or break your success. Poor little me, I had to give up something I really enjoyed. People are taking away my freedom to smoke when they won't let me smoke in their homes, restaurants. All my friends smoke. All of these are thoughts you are going to have to deal with. And here's the worst one: just one puff won't hurt. Yes, it will, and you need to have strategies to deal with them all.

Here are a few suggestions:

Do something, anything; get beyond the moment. Take a walk, call a friend, take a hot bath or shower, clean a closet, anything. Remember, millions of people who have quit have learned how to get past those thoughts, and you must learn to do it too.

Create a list of reasons you must quit; you'll be able to think of a dozen or so. Don't be afraid to read the list over and over again. Remember that the urge to use is short lived and will pass. It will become easier to put your heel in its forehead with each passing hour.

Create a mantra: the motto of your successful trip to quit using. "Hell no!" says it all in two easy to remember words. You can just use the initials HN in proper company or libraries.

Read the experiment and prove to yourself that a deep breath held for a while can have the same effect as a puff of you-know-what. It's not quite the same? Lie to yourself, play games with your mind: here's where a little deceit is okay. Just to get through the moment! Fly a kite, write a poem. Anything to win.

Create a rewards system—fund it with your savings.

A pack of smokes a day turns into ten bucks in the old sock. Five days of that runs into a great dinner, a movie, and small popcorn or half of a new pair of great walking shoes. Wait a minute, would that be $3,650 bucks a years? Youbetcha as they say in Minnesota. You're starting to talk a real vacation here.

Make your life space nicotine free. Car (under the car seat), cabin, boat, basement, favorite hiding place, old purses, suit jackets, overcoats, and the ledge above the garage door are all places that have housed half-empty packs of smokes that you might find at the wrong time. Don't forget matches, pipe cleaners, tobacco pouches, ashtrays, etc. "Scorched earth" means everything even remotely connected to nicotine goes into the "farewell forever" box to be disposed of on D-Day minus 1.

Remember it only hurts for a little while. Want to know something? Giving up nicotine addiction doesn't hurt at all unless you tell yourself it will. Actually, the pros say that by the time you have been nicotine free for a day, the carbon monoxide level in your blood goes down to normal as does your risk of heart attack within a couple weeks. Although quitting nicotine use can have its tough moments, it can be easy - and even fun - to 'fool' your own mind into getting past those moments. My sister tried many times to quit but never succeeded. Please be assured that dying of nicotine-induced cancer is much harder than kicking nicotine.

Two Days before D-Day

Make one more sweep of all known spaces where nicotine may have been stashed. Throw any newly found junk into the farewell forever box, take the box, render all material in it unusable, and dispose of it in the junk or garbage.

The last thing to go into your farewell forever box should be any nicotine products you were planning to use the next day. That's right. The next day—the day before you were going to quit, except that you just quit using nicotine a day earlier than you expected.

When you wake up on D Day, you will be able to truthfully tell yourself "I quit yesterday." The day before you were planning on quitting. You're already a day ahead!

Take a deep, deep breath and hold it, let it out slowly.

Don't be afraid to cheat your mind—it can even become fun; remember the tricks it has played on you. And this is all for a good purpose.

Congratulations, quitter!

Today's the day to take a walk around the closest lake unless you live in Duluth, Minnesota.

Go fishing with a non-nicotine-using friend.

Take many deep breaths and hold them. Repeat as needed.

Notice that strange smell? It's called "fresh air."

Please enjoy the rest of your life as a non-nicotine user; you've earned every deep breath of it!

Resources

1. Mayo Clinic Website: Nicotine Dependence
2. HHS Public Access: Nicotine Addiction NIHMSID NIHMS227888
    Neal L. Benowitz M.D. University of California
3. Medical News Today Website
4. Psychology Today Website: Nicotine https://www.psychologytoday.com/us/conditions/nicotine
5. Center for Tobacco Research and Education Website: Tobacco is Not Caffeine: Stanton A. Glantz PhD https://tobacco.ucsf.edu/nicotine-not-caffein
6. American Lung Association Website: E-cigarettes and Lung Health
    http://www.luna.ora/stop-smoking/smoking-facts/ e-cigarettes-and-lung health.html
7. Yale Medicine: Your Teen is Underestimating the Health Risks Of Vaping, by Kathleen Raven (Kathleen.Raven@yale.edu
8. Time Health: Why Juul Is At the Center of the FDA's E-Cigarette Investigation
    http://time.com/5413690/fda-iuul-investigation

About the Author

Doug Ewald lives in Minnetonka, Minnesota, with his wife of more than sixty years, Ginny. They are parents of six children, have eighteen grandchildren, and eleven great-grandchildren.

He holds bachelor and master's degrees in public health from the University of Minnesota.

Doug served four terms in the Minnesota House of Representatives. He was the founder of Ewald Consulting, a multiassociation management and government relations corporation based in St. Paul.

Twenty-three years after beginning to smoke and after many unsuccessful attempts to quit, he finally quit by using the methods described in this book. Twenty-two months after quitting, he completed the New York City Marathon, and sixteen other marathons followed. His daily habit of a morning walk/run, which started as a strategy for nicotine cessation, continues each morning "as long as it's above twenty-five degrees below zero."